APPLE CIDER VINEGAR

A Simple DIY Manual: How to Make Apple Cider Vinegar from Scraps in Few Minutes and Get Rid of Fat
Included: Over 15 Other Mind Blowing Health Benefits

SAMUEL MONALISA
Copyright@2018

COPYRIGHT

No part of this publication may be reproduced, distributed, or transmitted in any form or by any means, including photocopying, recording, or other electronic or mechanical methods, or by any information storage and retrieval system without the prior written permission of the publisher, except in the case of very brief quotations embodied in critical reviews and certain other noncommercial uses per-mitted by copyright law.

Samuel Monalisa

TABLE OF CONTENT

CHAPTER ONE 4
   INTRODUCTION 4
CHAPTER TWO 6
   HOW TO MAKE APPLE CIDER VINEGAR FROM SCRAPS...6
CHAPER THREE 11
   IMPORTANT NOTES 11
CHAPTER FOUR 13
   APPLE CIDER VINEGAR WEIGHT LOSS 13
CHAPTER FIVE 15
   BENEFITS AND USES OF APPLE CIDER VINEGAR 15
CHAPTER SIX 26
   PRECAUTIONS: HOW MUCH APPLE CIDER VINEGAR SHOULD YOU TAKE?...26
THE END...28

CHAPTER ONE

INTRODUCTION

The advantages of self-made apple cider vinegar can't be over emphasize, It's no secret us homesteader people are entire enthusiasts about the stuff—we use it for everything from cleaning, to cooking, to animal care and the whole lot in between. The fitness benefits of uncooked apple cider vinegar are totally impressive, too. But did you understand you can virtually make it barring any charges?

Samuel Monalisa

Really interesting, there are numerous extra complicated ways to make apple cider vinegar at home, but nowadays I'm gonna show you how to make it from apple scraps. I particularly like this approach since it allows me to use the apples for different stuff (like yummy self-made applesauce) whilst nevertheless making a treasured product from the "waste". I additionally like it due to the fact it's loopy easy. And I'm lazy.

CHAPTER TWO

HOW TO MAKE APPLE CIDER VINEGAR FROM SCRAPS

Items needed:

1. Apple peelings or cores
2. Sugar (1 tablespoon per one cup of water)
3. Water
4. Glass jar (a quart is a splendid area to start, but you can without a doubt make large quantities, too.)

Instructions

a. Fill the glass jar ¾ of the way with apple peels and cores.

b. Stir the sugar into the water till it's typically dissolved, and pour over the apple scraps till they are totally covered. (Leave a few inches of room at the pinnacle of the jar.)

c. Cover loosely (I suggest a coffee filter or cloth scrap secured with a rubber band) and set in a warm, darkish place for around two weeks.

d. You can supply it a stir each few days, if you like. If any brownish/greyish scum develops on the top, clearly skim it off.

e. Once two weeks has passed, pressure the scraps from the liquid.

Apple Cider Vinegar

f. *At this point, my vinegar normally has a pleasantly candy apple cider smell, however is nonetheless missing that beautiful tang.*

g. *Discard the scraps (or feed them to your chickens!), and set the strained liquid aside for every other 2-4 weeks.*

h. *You'll recognize your apple cider vinegar is complete as soon as it has that unmistakable vinegary smell and taste. If it's no longer quite there yet, virtually permit it to take a seat a whilst longer.*

i. *Once you are completely happy with the taste of your vinegar, simply cap and save in the fridge as long as you like. It won't go bad.*

j. If a gelatinous blob develops on the pinnacle of your vinegar, congratulations! You have created a vinegar "mother". This mom can be use to jump-start future vinegar batches. You can get rid of it and keep it separately, however I commonly simply allow mine to flow around in the vinegar as I shop it.

k. Use your selfmade vinegar simply like you would store-bought vinegar– for cooking, cleaning and the whole lot in between!

About keeping and pickling with home made vinegar: It's usually endorsed that you do NOT use home made vinegar for any type of preservation. In order to make sure the safety of your home canned products, you need a vinegar with a acetic acid degree of 5%. Since most of us don't have a way to take a look at the stages of our selfmade vinegar, it's quality just to pass the usage of it for canning or preserving– better secure than sorry!

Samuel Monalisa

CHAPER THREE

IMPORTANT NOTES

If your household doesn't like peels in their homemade applesauce, this is the perfect way to maintain them from going to waste.

It's perfectly pleasant to use scraps from barely bruised or browned apples for your vinegar. However avoid the use of rotten or moldy fruit.

Don't have sufficient apple scraps for a full batch? No problem– just acquire your scraps in the freezer until you have ample for a full jar.

Since we're using the peels for this recipe, I fairly suggest starting with natural apples to avoid any pesticides or chemical residues.

Apple Cider Vinegar

You ought to use honey (affiliate) in place of the sugar in this recipe if you virtually desired too. However, the use of honey will slow down the method a bit.

Also, hold in idea the really useful organisms will be consuming the sugar for the duration of the fermentation process, so there'll be little to no sugar left in the closing product.

You can make any extent of vinegar you like—my first batch was once in a quart jar, but now I've graduated to a gallon jar. *a-hem*

Looking for something new and interesting to make with your DIY apple cider vinegar? Try this DIY home made gatorade.

You can simply scan with different fruit scraps too— pears and peaches especially.

CHAPTER FOUR

APPLE CIDER VINEGAR WEIGHT LOSS

Apple cider vinegar can assist you lose weight. Previously in 8000 BC, the Egyptians made used of ACV for weight loss. This age-old fitness remedy is made from the fermented juice of apples and helps decrease blood pressure and cholesterol, treats acne and sore throat, and fights cancer. In this book, you will understand how ACV aids weight loss, how to include it in your diet, and other health advantages of ingesting apple cider vinegar.

The apple cider vinegar diet

If you lose weight quickly, your body will oblige you by kicking in mechanisms to make it more in all likelihood this weight will slip lower back on in no time. But if you can be patient and do now not expect immediate results, your fat cells will alter to their new measurement more willingly and not insist on contributing on your waistline. The apple cider vinegar food plan is best for this.

CHAPTER FIVE

BENEFITS AND USES OF APPLE CIDER VINEGAR

Low In Calories

Apple cider vinegar is low in calories. One teaspoon of apple cider vinegar provides only 1 calorie.

Hence, you will not be at the threat of adding too many energy to your diet. And the fewer the energy you consume, the much less prone you will be to shop the greater energy as fat.

Lowers Serum Lipid Levels

Scientists designed an scan to report the consequences of ACV on complete cholesterol, serum triglyceride, lipid peroxidation, and antioxidant levels. They determined that mice supplemented with ACV had developed higher immunity, lower serum lipid levels, improved antioxidant levels, and inhibited lipid peroxidation. All the parameters used in this find out about are at once or not directly associated to weight loss and point out that drinking apple cider vinegar can assist enhance your normal health.

Burns Fat

There are various studies which established that taking apple cider vinegar has shown an amplify in fat burning and limit in fat accumulation.

"As per study, when overweight contributors have been given day by day dosage of apple cider vinegar over 12 weeks, they have determined discount in stomach fat, waist length, weight and blood triglycerides

Enhance Metabolism

Decreased metabolism can regularly lead to fat accumulation and weight gain. Many fad diets and industrial drugs can regularly reduce your metabolism once you end them which is the predominant purpose for speedy weight gain. The acids found in apple cider vinegar build-up digestion and metabolism.

"As per a find out about conducted on rats, the acetic acid existing in apple cider vinegar has extended AMPK enzyme. This enzyme is helpful in increasing fat burning, limit stomach fat storage and liver fat.

Makes you experience full

When ACV is ate up earlier than meals, the pectin existing in it suppresses you urge for food and leaves you feel full for a longer time. This helps to control starvation pangs and stop binge consuming – one of the pleasant ways to manipulate wait reap overtime.

"In a find out about conducted in 2005, the members were given varying tiers of apple cider vinegar and carbohydrates in the structure of white bread. The individuals who had most apple cider vinegar felt fuller and extra satiated than others

Contains Beneficial Probiotics

80% of immune device is supported by way of a healthy gut. Our intestine carries proper and bad bacteria, when this stability is disturbed it can exhibit a direct effect on our immune system. Improving intestine health reduces the irritation and prevents obesity. ACV is one of the fantastic probiotics which carries many top bacterial strains.

"As per the find out about published with the aid of Journal of Clinical Investigation, probiotic micro organism can be helpful in weight loss and stopping obesity. Several different studies have additionally tested the same.

Improves Better Sleep
Apple cider vinegar when blended with some honey becomes an notable remedy for insomnia. Lack of proper sleep regularly increases ghrelin a hormone which is responsible for stimulating starvation pangs. Apple cider vinegar plays some trick on our brain for a good sleep that regulates both hunger and our stress hormones.
"In numerous research work, like the published one in International Journal of Obesity, people with bad sleep and stress less likely to reap weight loss dreams.

Apple cider vinegar soothes a sore throat

As soon as you experience the prickle of a sore throat, rent germ-busting apple cider vinegar to assist head off the contamination at the pass. Turns out, most germs can't survive in the acidic surroundings vinegar creates. Just combine 1/4 cup apple cider vinegar with 1/4 cup warm water and gargle each hour or so.

Apple cider vinegar treats hiccups

Take a teaspoonful of apple cider vinegar; its sour taste ought to cease a hiccup in its tracks. One teen took the hiccup remedy in addition and created a lollipop that includes apple cider vinegar, which she says "cancels out the message to hiccup" through overstimulating the nerves in the throat responsible for the spasms. (Carryout more research on how to take an apple cider vinegar bath to gain even more of its benefits.)

Apple cider vinegar clears a stuffy nose

Next time you're stuffed up from a cold, seize the apple cider vinegar. It incorporates potassium, which thins mucus; and the acetic acid in it prevents germ growth, which may want to contribute to nasal congestion. Mix a teaspoon of apple cider vinegar in a glass of water and drink to assist sinus drainage.

Apple cider vinegar used for whitening teeth

Gargle with apple cider vinegar in the morning. The vinegar helps put off stains, whiten teeth, and kill micro organism in your mouth and gums. Brush as typical after you gargle. You can also brush your teeth with baking soda as soon as a week to assist put off stains and whiten your teeth; use it simply as you would toothpaste. You can additionally use salt as an alternative toothpaste. If your gums start to feel raw, swap to brushing with salt each and every different day.

Apple cider vinegar ease dead night leg cramps

Leg cramps can regularly be a signal that you're low in potassium. Since one of the many apple cider vinegar benefits is that it's excessive in potassium, one domestic remedy says mixing 1 teaspoon honey and tablespoons apple cider vinegar to a glass of warm water and drink to stop night-time leg cramps. Of course, through the time you stroll to the kitchen to put the drink together, your cramp is likely to be history—but possibly that's the point.

Heals Poison Ivy

ACV is a herbal remedy that can assist soothe an itchy poison ivy rash. This is because it contains potassium, which may additionally help decrease the swelling associated with poison ivy. Try applying a teaspoon without delay to the pores and skin a few times per day until it is healed.

Treats Growths or Warts

Have you tried to get rid of a growth or wart and it won't go away? Make a cotton ball and soak it in ACV, making use of without delay to the wart and overlaying with a bandage overnight. Though it may additionally take a while, repeating this a few times can cause the wart to eventually fall right off.

Use as a Natural Deodorant

The armpits are a great breeding spot for bacteria, which can lead to a worsening of physique odor. ACV possesses powerful antibacterial homes and makes an wonderful natural deodorant. One of the easiest apple cider vinegar uses is to dab a bit on your fingers and follow below your palms to assist neutralize smell and hold you smelling fresh.

Kills Bugs and Fleas

If your dog or cat can't give up scratching themselves, ditch the chemical-laden flea killers and attempt this natural remedy instead. Add equal components water and apple cider vinegar to a spray bottle and observe to the fur as soon as per day until fleas are gone. You can also strive making your personal homemade worm spray and making use of to your skin to battle off pesky insects.

Protect Against Seasonal Allergies

Many people use apple cider vinegar as a herbal remedy for seasonal allergies. The healthful bacteria determined in ACV may also promote immunity and aid healthful lymphatic drainage to kick seasonal sniffles and allergies to the curb. Try to drink two tablespoons diluted in water subsequent time your hypersensitive reactions are performing up.

CHAPTER SIX

PRECAUTIONS: HOW MUCH APPLE CIDER VINEGAR SHOULD YOU TAKE?

Although apple cider vinegar consumption is healthful and secure for most people, taking large amounts can lead to some terrible effects on health. Apple cider vinegar aspect results encompass erosion of tooth enamel, burning of the throat or pores and skin and lowered tiers of potassium.

Be positive to always dilute apple cider vinegar in water as an alternative of ingesting it straight to prevent terrible side effects. You ought to also begin with a low dose and work your way up to verify your tolerance.

If you're taking blood sugar medications, discuss to your doctor before the usage of apple cider vinegar. Because ACV may also help reduce blood sugar levels, you may also need to alter your dosage of diabetes medicines to stop hypoglycemia symptoms.

Finally, while there are a extensive vary of apple cider vinegar uses, it shouldn't be seen as a rapid restoration or therapy when it comes to your health. Instead, it have to be paired with a nutritious weight loss plan and wholesome way of life to in reality see results.

Samuel Monalisa

THE END

Samuel Monalisa

www.ingramcontent.com/pod-product-compliance
Lightning Source LLC
Chambersburg PA
CBHW031518210526
45464CB00007B/2973